Starting Over

Learning to Live in a Healthy World Created by You

Darrin Eaddy

FORWARD

As I change my lifestyle to embrace and walk in health, I have had to do the work of researching what health means, how to achieve it, and what inhibited me from embracing it naturally. It was the latter work of understanding my own habits and broken mindset that has taken the most energy, resources, and acceptance of my own shortcomings.

It has been my experience that most of us want to walk in health. Still, we simply may not have the healthy attitudes and self-esteem that is necessary to fuel the change that a new lifestyle requires. It is for those of us who need frank discussion regarding healthy behaviors, the mirror placed in front of faces to reveal our own limitations, and at times a cheerleader with the proper words and resources that Darrin Eaddy wrote this book.

Mr. Eaddy does not write this book in the western tradition where thoughts and ideas are presented linearly and build toward a climatic conceptual conclusion. Rather, this book is a conversation, reflecting his lifelong career in fitness and health promotion. Use his voice as a tool to help you adopt the attitudes, behaviors and beliefs necessary to move into a life true wealth—health of your body, mind, and spirit.

Following are 30 days of reflective thought each with an action step that you can take toward living a healthier lifestyle. I encourage you to take each step one moment, day, week, or month at a time. Remember, half of the joy and benefit of living a healthy lifestyle is in the journey!

With you in the walk,

Dr. Regina E. Wragg

ACKNOWLEDGEMENTS

I want to thank God for vision and purpose in my life.

Having the partnership of good friends made this journey so much more meaningful and important. I thank Courtney Black and Dr. Regina Wragg for their contributions to this book to make it a success.

INTRODUCTION

To change your life you must first change yourself. With this understanding to have a better life, you must first know what kind of life you want. A friend of mine told me that we live in a life of grey because we are too afraid to live in a world of black and white. I believe what she says is true to a certain extent-- we no longer have a clear picture of what is black and white, up and down, or truly right and truly wrong. It all has been shaded for us by society's values and programmed moral compass.

There is not much that I can say in this book that has not been said before in other books, on YouTube, or in the news. Still, I am a man who more than 20 years ago began to make a career of fitness with a blurred understanding of what fitness and health truly meant. In the beginning, I knew that a healthy body could accomplish almost anything, and for a time, I was right but only as it applied to myself.

I thought that I had a complete understanding of what the mind and body could do, but I never really knew that I was missing something in the equation. Over time, I learned that the missing element was something that was a part of me and that I was always tapping into—spirit. At one point, I placed most of my life's success on my own skill or simple dumb luck, but never on faith. Even though I had faith, I never thought it played a true part in shaping my life. I believed all choices were mine and that all consequences, both good and bad, were results of my own doing.

What changed my life was the fact that I accepted that I was called to help others. My calling, should you ask, is that I am a personal trainer and fitness consultant. It is a simple enough job, and to most people, it is no big deal. But when you know God has placed a purpose on your life to not only help people physically but to also help his people from a spiritual position as well, the simplicity of the job all but disappears. Now I walk the path of mind, body, and spirit. This path better shapes an understanding of what complete health is truly all about. So, I have started over in my life adding spirit to my mind and body so that I can better assist the people I am called on to help.

I ask everyone who chooses to read this book to start over and walk a life with a positive outlook, expectation of new beginnings, and a full understanding of what health truly means. With an understanding of mind, body and spirit, you then have an understanding of true health.

Darrin Eaddy

TABLE OF CONTENTS

YOU HAVE TO MAKE A CHOICE TO LIVE A BETTER, HEALTHIER LIFE.

It sounds so simple, but the first step is wanting it. It's a mental step, and a big one at that. Do you want it? There is no physical exertion what so ever required to make this decision, but it seems like the hardest part of the process. Make up your mind to do it…then do it.

To have a better life, you must change your behavior so you can realize new feelings and understandings about yourself. The only constant about life is change. Things can change day by day, and taking note of the daily changes will help you see life much clearer. How well do you adapt to change? Are you even willing and prepared to adapt?

Your belief must come from your faith and it must also come from your trust that you want the best for yourself. You shouldn't sabotage you success! You must pursue your health and happiness with drive, motivation and passion!

Today's Action Step: Write "I Choose Health" on adhesive slips and post them all over your home to remind you to choose health.

MAKE A LIST OF THE PROS AND CONS ABOUT LIVING A HEALTHY LIFE.

Write it out! What matters to you when it comes to health? What are your goals? What do they look like on paper? What are the good things about being healthy? What are the bad things about not getting healthy? Which list looks better? What stops you from getting healthy? What would motivate you? These are things that you should ask yourself and answer accordingly.

If you were to create a list of all the things that distract you from moving toward your goals of health, it could possibly be a long list of things that are both inside and outside of your control. Here is where the Serenity Prayer becomes your friend. For example, if not having time to exercise is on your list of what keeps you from getting to your goals, then ask yourself how much time do you spend watching TV per week? (And TV is just ONE well known distracter!)

When starting over and deciding what to do, the thing you need the most is education. So the next questions you may ask are "what am I supposed to do and how do I do it?"

Today's Action Step: Write down your daily actions for 3 days. Include what you do and how long you do it. After you have your list, make a trade-off; for example, if you watch an hour of TV, rededicate 30 minutes to exercise.

HEALTH IS A FORM OF STRENGTH JUST LIKE HAVING A COLLEGE DEGREE OR GOOD JOB.

When people peruse their goals in life, what steps do they take?   Everybody knows that if you fail to plan, you plan to fail, right? We look at things like what type of education we will need, what type of job skills we need to procure, and with whom we need to be friends in the office. (Don't pretend like you've never thought about it.)

You have a vision of what you want, but your vision must be manifested into an action plan--you need both! A vision without action is just an illusion, and action without vision is just plain confusion. Ask yourself, "why do I want these things?" and "how do I get them?" These same questions can be posed to your health or lack of it. But if your life starts and ends with you and you say that you want a better life, then you first have to want health. But do you really want it? Meaning, are you able to develop a vision and action plan for your health? If you are not, are you willing to get help to do so?

Today's Action Step: Prepare your day with health in mind, such as "do I have water?," "what are my food choices for today?," or "when will I exercise?" Some people may find planning works best the day before while others may find that preparing for the day should happen the morning of. Seek help planning the number of calories and frequency of your meals if you need it, and don't begin a new exercise routine before consulting a qualified professional.

WHAT VALUES DO YOU PLACE ON YOUR LIFE?

We are taught to change our life for the better by adding simple principles and values that we will use to govern what we do. However, none of those original principles involve health. Society teaches us that money, homes, cars, and land are all valuable and that we should spend our lives in pursuit of these things. But we can die trying because health is not part of what society teaches is valuable.

What is your personal value? What are you worth to you? How do you feel about you? Do you take the time to appreciate who you are and what God has given you? Is your life important enough to take care of yourself for you? We are self-destructive people because we choose to kill ourselves for other people or other things, but we don't sacrifice enough time for our own well-being and sanity. WE DIE in the constant pursuit of other people's happiness.

You must see your happiness in your mind's eye and have a clear picture of what happiness looks like to you. How you achieve your happiness comes later, but for now, just know what you want for your healthy life. It all starts with a vision. As stated previously, a vision without action is just an illusion, action without a vision is just plain confusion, but a vision combined with action can give you a life transfusion!

To start over you must push yourself to get past the things that limit your success like fear, shame, approval from others, lack of discipline, and lack of understanding. These are just obstacles to overcome. This is just your proving ground of battles to be won. Know that none of these obstacles actually stop your goal of living a healthy lifestyle. They only provide you with opportunities to develop strength on your journey!

Today's Action Step: Write down your fears so you can have a clear picture of where your struggle comes from. Don't dwell on the list, but get them out of your head and onto paper. As you walk in your commitment to your health, revisit your list periodically and take note of how you've grown past your fears.

KNOW WHO YOU ARE AND WHAT VALUES MAKE UP YOUR CHARACTER.

Watch your thoughts they become words. Watch your words, they become actions, watch your actions they become habit. Watch your habits, they become character. Watch your character, it becomes your destiny. - Lao Tzu

How you shape your life will come down to your value structure. If you believe stealing is wrong then your values will not allow you to steal. It's as simple as that.

To make the changes that will become a permanent part of your life, you must first have a better understanding of your personal behavior. How you deal with your life will help you understand your short comings. Most people are not aware of some of the things they do. So from their own perspective, nothing is wrong, but to other people, it seems like they have big problems.

What is your personal image? What do you like about yourself that brings a smile to your face when you wake up each day? Can you pinpoint your strengths, and do you know what your weaknesses are? These are just more questions to help identify who you are and why you want to change. If you don't have enough things in your life that makes you happy about yourself then you know change must come.

Today's Action Step: Ask yourself, "who am I" and "what makes me a good person?"

THE VALUES YOU CHOOSE WILL PAINT THE PICTURE YOUR LIFE WILL FOLLOW.

What are your top ten values and which of these values would you apply to your healthy lifestyle? Your values will help you shape your motivation about being healthy or not. What's your motivation? What are you doing to live this motivation? Do you do it to feel better? Look better? Be better?

Throughout life, we are taught certain life lessons that govern us as we grow, but how we use those life lessons dictate what we do and ultimately who we become. So what if certain life lessons are left out such as how to eat the right foods or how to actively live a healthy lifestyle? Who is to blame? Would you blame your parents for not being healthy? Would you? The truth is your body is just that-- your body. No one else has your body (unless you have a doppelgänger, then that's creepy, and we're not talking to you). While genetics may have their way from time to time, it's still not considered a constant. Again, YOUR health solely relies on YOU.

Starting over is looking past the wrong decisions and looking for the right ones that will change the way we live our lives. These right choices will help change the world we live in by establishing health as more valuable than positions or wealth. Having a healthy mind leads to a healthy body, which leads to a healthy life. So, let's begin a new life by starting over.

Today's Action Step: Make a list of your motivations for living a healthy lifestyle.

CHOOSE YOUR VALUES CAREFULLY; YOUR LIFESTYLE WILL DEPEND ON IT.

We live in a world of viewpoints that society has set up as guidelines. And as unfair or unfounded as they may be, we judge ourselves and others by these guidelines. For example, societal guidelines say success is having a nice car or house, having lots of money, or just being famous. Still, is this the picture of success that aligns with your self-determined values, vision, and action plan? What is your worth? How is it measured? Who is measuring it? I can bet that one of those previously mentioned societal guidelines is at the core of your personal value structure.

You can't start at the end; you must start from the beginning. Your life starts with being healthy and it should be the first education one should have as a core value and understanding. Some of us don't view health as a measure of success, so it is not high on our list of values.

Today's Action Step: It's no secret that most of us are creatures of habit. You live a life of habits and routines. What part of those habits and routines positively improve the quality of your life? Take a moment to list your daily, weekly, and monthly habits and routines. Evaluate if and how your habits and routines add value to your life.

EDUCATE YOURSELF ON WHAT A TRUE HEALTHY LIFESTYLE LOOKS LIKE—MIND, BODY, AND SPIRIT.

Stay in the now, but change for the future. We can only do what we know; how we respond to situations or how we even answer questions is based on the knowledge we have available to us. So without new education, we will continue to make the same mistakes.

A healthy lifestyle is not what you see on TV with those heavily advertised and sponsored weight loss programs or infomercials designed to get into your head and wallet. It's about connecting your mind, body, and spirit together to create a new way of living your life.

To do something new, you have to learn something new. Why must you learn something new? Simply put, you have bad habits that prevent you from improving. Most of us just settle into our lives and give up on making changes. Usually that will lead to a lot of medical, financial, or health problems because we let so many things go wrong before we decide to do it right Now that you have started to educate yourself on what's important to achieve a healthy lifestyle, you must first choose where to start. There is a lot of information on just about everything, so take your time to break things down.

Today's Action Step: Spend some time with a personal trainer or fitness coach or buy a book on basic health to gain an educated perspective on what your healthy lifestyle should be.

NEVER LET GLUTTONY BE YOUR DOWNFALL; LEARN TO CONTROL IT.

To be born in America is a joy and a curse. This is the land of abundance and opportunity. We live in a supersized world where we continue to consume more food, take in more sugar, and exercise less. You can do anything you want in this world. But as you can see, looking at the state of obesity, depression, and drug abuse, achieving self-discipline is a must-- it's a matter of survival.

To receive tangible or non-tangible things in life, we must first desire them. We have an undeniable craving for the pleasures of this world, but we have to ask ourselves, "what pushes us to this point in our lives to want so much than we ever need?" We are slaves to our senses. We don't want to admit it, but we follow our senses like animals and we do so without thought. We let what we see, feel, and taste control what we do.

So where do you have examples of how to discipline yourself? Why would you want to? The truth is if you can't be disciplined with your eating and exercise routine, everything else will be just as hard. Being able to resist our urges to overeat just because we can, find a shortcut instead of working through to a solution, or to want something just because we see it are some of the biggest transformations we can have on the inside.

Today's Action Step: Honestly reflect on your fitness and nutrition regimen. What does self-discipline look like for you?

YOUR LIFESTYLE MUST HAVE MEANING TO YOU.

What does it mean to you? Being able to help yourself is a major accomplishment. You have to identify the problem, isolate the problem, and then seek a resolution to your problem. Most people won't make themselves vulnerable enough to know that they are on the brink of crisis. For the average person, knowing where you have a problem and then being able to and come up with a solution shows an advanced level of honesty, acceptance, and maturity.

Do you know why you want to have a healthy life? Can you feel a new beginning in your spirit? Does it call to you to make changes? Do you dream about the new you? Can you almost taste how close it is to be the person you know you can be? That my friend is desire! That special feeling you have inside that pushes you forward. It can see you through the bad times and help you elevate the good.

You must write down how you are going to get there. You are at the beginning stages of having a system. Now you can track your progress because all the components of your success are beginning to shine through and your confidence is beginning to grow within yourself. Now that you have the confidence, you have to keep going. Now your dream is becoming a reality. Piece by piece, it will all come together.

Today's Action Step: What are some of your problem areas that prevent you from living a healthy lifestyle that can benefit you in ways beyond the physical gains? Really think about what's holding you back, isolate it, and make a plan to defeat and resolve it! And there you have it — you will be on your way to making your first change toward improving your life!

YOU CAN MAKE CHOICES THAT IMPROVE YOUR DAY.

Discipline yourself to take care of your body in a way that makes it healthy and strong.

Have you ever been in a group project? Have you ever had the one person in the group that never pulled their fair share of the load? What happened? It caused everybody else in the group to step up and account for what was lacking to ensure success; or that part of the project went lacking, and everybody's grade or performance record suffered in some part.

Your body works the same way in that sometimes your overall quality becomes affected due to what is found to be lacking. We are comprised of mind, body, and spirit. Each of these is interdependent on the other in order to help you function. What you feed into most is what governs you. (Take a moment and let that marinate because we will talk about that some more.)

How you eat will also give you a level of discipline that will better control the life you lead. If you place value on your health, it will give you a different perspective on what kind of meaning your life will have. Eating healthy takes a level of discipline. That discipline will carry over to other parts of your life.

Today's Action Step: Add something fitness or health related to your daily routine such as reading an article, doing an exercise, or trying a healthy recipe (see the appendix for healthy eating ideas). Commit to doing it!

NEVER MAKE AN EXCUSE FOR BEING LAZY! SLOTH CAN CREEP IN AND BECOME A WAY OF LIFE.

Now the biggest road block to fulfilling our destiny of a healthy lifestyle that is affecting not only the adults but also our children is the level in which we choose to be non-productive. To put it in layman's terms, we are a lazy bunch of people! Now I don't mean that to cover all aspects of our lives, but I do apply it toward our pursuit of a healthy lifestyle. Simply put, it is easy to be lazy. There's a type of freedom to giving in and ultimately giving up. It takes the burden of expectation and accountability off of us. Society has manufactured this "giving up" sense of freedom that allows it to be okay to be non-active and complacent. This laziness is allowed through freedom of choice.

The constant advancement of technology has simplified life to the point of no effort in which to pursue anything that matters to your life's well-being. Examples of this have evolved over the years from the TV remote, to the microwave, and now to YouTube and Google where knowledge (and opinion) of everything is at your fingertips. We have been reduced to a level of inactivity and low productivity that is appalling to witness by someone who is concerned and conscious of the community's health.

So let's put all of this into perspective-- you only have one life. If you waste it, you will not get another. But if it was just you wasting your life and it did not affect anyone else's well-being, then it would just be between you and God. However, you wasting your life away is not an isolated event in our world. Our individual actions affect the people all around us. From low productivity at work to poor examples of healthy lifestyles at home, our lack to make and act in productive choices affects our families and those around us and not just ourselves. All of the mis-informed and ill-made choices add up people, and now we find ourselves in the state we are in today.

Think of your healthy lifestyle as making a contribution to this world. We never see our lack of activity or poor eating as a part of a world destroying decision. Having an unhealthy lifestyle is like an undiagnosed cancer that kills so slowly that you don't notice until it is too late.

Today's Action Step: Make it your intention to take notice of where you are being lazy. If you are out shopping, park in the rear of the lot. When you are walking around a multilevel building, take the stairs. While watching television, do some cardio or strength training. Make activity a choice!

KNOW YOU! STUDY YOU! ASK YOURSELF QUESTIONS TO BE CLEAR ON WHO YOU ARE.

Most people hide who they are, and they're masters of it. They keep themselves apart from the rest of the world, and they never get to the point of letting people see their true selves. They live a lie that they let other people buy into.

While mastering others is strength of sorts, mastering yourself is a sign of true power. Know that you are powerful! You can't hide your weight or the energy you give off. So why try? If you're unhappy about the way you look or feel, then change it-- because you want to and because you can!

Today's Action Step: Make a list of who you are and who you project to others. Ask some trusted friends to share with you what you exhibit to them. Be willing to accept their truth. How does your intended projection align with what you actually display?

SEE YOURSELF IN A POSITIVE WAY, AND THAT WILL ALLOW OTHERS TO SEE YOU THAT WAY, TOO.

Whether you think you can or can't...You're right.

Most people never take the time to address themselves like they address other people. We seem to always make a judgment about someone else's life, and we never get around to judging or evaluating our own.

We forget that we live in glass houses (...dusty glass houses at that!), and in that same token, we praise things in others that we too could or do possess if we were to give ourselves the proper attention. I don't know if you have seen the ads from a popular retailer in which they ask the question, "what does your coat say about you?" In the ads, the people unashamedly and publicly yell out what their favorite coats say about them. (YouTube this commercial!) The things they yell out are positive things that they believe to be true about themselves. As funny as it is, it asks the question, "what is your state of health saying about you?" and in essence, "what are you saying about you?"

Knowing is half the battle. If knowledge is power then your lack of education about your body and what it takes to be and stay healthy impairs your ability to move forward in life. In layman's terms: if you knew better, you would do better.

Today's Action Step: Write down at least one positive thing about yourself every day. If you run out of items, it is okay to rewrite something you stated previously. The point is to reinforce your value and to have an encouraging moment in your daily life.

ARE YOU HEALTHY OR NOT-- THAT IS THE QUESTION? HONESTY IS THE BEST POLICY.

NEVER LIE. And if you're one of the few that do it…then at least never lie to yourself about happiness — your own happiness! If you aren't living your own reality then whose myth are you?

How you feel about yourself can manifest itself in a negative or positive way in your life. These feelings can dictate the actions you do and don't take. Remember, we are mind, body, and spirit. Having an unhealthy lifestyle can limit your choices and affect the overall quality of your life.

 A healthy life is a certain walk just like someone who lives a Christian life has a Christian walk. As, we are taught to guard our eyes and ears and most importantly our hearts from things that might make us fall off of the track or distract us. Your journey in fitness has the same concepts-- guard your eyes (from the hot sign at the ohhhh so tempting donut shop), guard your hands (from grabbing junk food at the store), and most importantly guard your mouth from consuming all that is detrimental to your health! (Can all the Saints in the fried chicken line after church say amen!) It's all in fun, but in all seriousness, what you do matters to your body. What you eat, how you exercise, and getting proper rest can become life habits.

The only thing constant is change--LIFE IS CHANGE. You can change your life! Your body is one of the things over which you do have control. You can look at your body as your personal platform of growth and education. If you can change your body, you can change your life and anything else. You're like your own science experiment (no Jedi mind trick folks). You can't predict tomorrow, but you can predict what you eat tomorrow. You can predict what you'll look like three months from now, and you can control how hard you will work out to get there. Control the controllable-- your body and how you feel in the skin you're in is controllable. Are you happy now?

Today's Action Step: Do your check list. Look in the mirror and write down what you love and what you'd like to change about your physical form.

NEVER LET PRIDE OR ENVY LIMIT YOUR ABILITY TO SEE THE BIGGER PICTURE WHEN IT COMES TO YOUR HEALTH.

Your pride will make you believe you have it all under control. Because of your pride, you will not think to ask for help, or even worse, refuse help when it is offered. Your pride will allow you to accept being unhealthy, and this self-destructive mindset will attack your spirit as well.

Sometimes we see the life we lead through other people's glasses. What I mean by that is we try to live someone else's life. We want to have what they have, live like they live, and we, in essence, want to become them. But when it doesn't work out (and it never does because we can never be another person), we have resentment and sometimes even hate.

Don't hate, re-evaluate. Don't let envy destroy the dream you have for yourself.

As we grow, we gain more clarity of our purpose and true happiness. God has a path for you and will give you the wisdom and courage to want things for yourself without looking for greener pastures. He makes no mistakes, nor does He set us up for failure. The choice is always ours. So you must believe your life is just as important as someone else's.

Today's Action Step: What is your vision of purpose and happiness? How does achieving your health goals influence your vision?

MAKE A PLAN THAT KEEPS YOU ACCOUNTABLE FOR YOUR LIFE.

Your life is about you-- how you feel, how you think and what you want. If what you want is to start over and add more value to your life, your body has all the potential you need to be the person you dream about being and to see your life and appearance transform before you. The world that you encounter during the journey is the magic that will shape you into the person you want to be!

What makes us different than other life forms is our ability to make mental changes and not just physical ones (and you thought it was just the opposable thumb!). We can look at our lives and see if we are improving or not improving and adjust accordingly. The world around us will always set the tone of what you do or don't do. If you can have the ability to think outside of the box, then you can change the world in which you live. Become the change you want to see in the world. Heck; become the change you want to see in the mirror!

Today's Action Step: Decide on two things that you can track about your change — one physical and one mental. For example, measuring your waistline or calf circumference can be ways to track your physical progress. Keeping a log where you briefly jot how you feel when you get up, before and after meals, or at the end of the day can be methods of gauging your mental changes.

LIVING A HEALTHY LIFE IS NOT A RACE-- YOU MUST HAVE PATIENCE TO LEARN WHAT WORKS FOR YOU.

Take it one meal at a time, one day at a time, and one foot in front of the other. It's not a race-- it's a journey. The only deadlines you have are the ones you set for yourself. No matter how fast or slow you go, you're still miles ahead of every person who hasn't even started. Do you!

It is said that imitation is the highest form of flattery, but not when it comes to fitness. Your body is YOUR body. Most of the time, we educate ourselves on health and fitness based off of what other people have done in the past. We imitate other people's success while never learning what our personal success looks like because we think if we don't have what they have (in body, resources or relationships),we have failed.

Today's Action Step: Pick a fitness plan and commit to it for thirty days (mark it off on a calendar). Use your goals that you wrote previously to measure your success. Remember, stick to it for 30 days before you tweak your plan!

CHOOSE A HEALTHY LIFE IN THE SAME FASHION YOU CHOOSE A FINANCIAL OR EDUCATIONAL ONE.

Being rich or being poor—each is a lifestyle and can bring out a certain amount of joy or pain. Still, neither guarantees how your life will turn out. You can go from being rich to poor or from poor to rich, but it all comes down to the journey. What did you gain or learn along the way to meeting your goals? Who did you meet that added wisdom and joy to your journey? Half of the fun is in the journey; the other half is in celebrating both large and small success. Achieving a healthy lifestyle is a journey that begins in the mind.

Living a healthy lifestyle will change your view on what you will and will not accept in your life. You will let the good things in and keep the bad things out. This principle can apply to all parts of your life. The principle of keeping what benefits you in and what harms you out won't be limited to the kitchen table. Learning to discipline your body teaches you to discipline your mind, and both are quite rewarding to your soul. A healthy lifestyle changes your view not only of what you will put in your body but also the activities and relationships that fill your life. When you began to expect and condition yourself to bring out the best in you, you won't settle for anything or anyone who doesn't.

Today's Action Step: Learn how to choose the right things for your life from a positive stand point. Review your words and actions from the previous day. Was there any point in time where you acted or accepted less than your best? What could you have done instead? Can you recall encouraging the best in someone else?

YOU CAN'T EXPECT YOUR MIND TO WORK RIGHT IF YOU DON'T HAVE THE RIGHT THINGS WITH WHICH TO WORK.

It may be hard to believe, but the average person is taught to fail. Our society based on consumerism wants you to live a life of mental slavery and control. Allowing an external entity (like music, TV, or your coveted leader) to think for you while not thinking for yourself is the best way to control your behavior and direction. So where would you get the mindset to live a positive life if you don't know what positive looks like for yourself? You have to be taught.

How many people really know how they are supposed to look or how they are supposed to feel? The average person has no real concept of health or what the body does to get healthy. We only know that we either feel good or we feel bad, and that my friends may be the extent of our understanding. With these types of limitations, people will continue to struggle with living a healthy lifestyle.

Our image of health is based on TV. What we see is how it is supposed to be. We see health in extreme spectrums — small frame and thin appearance to highly athletic with a physique of a God. These images are not the reality. A very small percentage of the population of the United States actually works out. Without learning what a physically active life looks like, you will never reach a level of activity to get that TV look that you see on every magazine and billboard.

Health is a very important part of life and people simply are not paying any attention to it on the level they should. If you can learn to see your world through a positive outlook, then life simply changes for the better. There is no down side to a healthy body. It should be at the forefront of all company heads before they consider hiring any employee. Being overweight or obese is causing more illness related to deaths and decreased quality of life than anything else. We have social standards that tell us not to drink and drive, wear our seatbelts, and have insurance, but it is okay to be unhealthy? Where are the standards resonating with physical fitness and nutrition?

Today's Action Step: Write your own health standard and place it in plain view (around your home, your work, or email signature). Examples could be "Don't eat while distracted," "Exercise today and every day," or "Eat more veggies."

NEVER LET ANGER OR GREED DRIVE YOUR DESIRE.

There is a certain truth to life that we know but won't fully acknowledge. There are many things in life that will go wrong, and there are many things in life that will go right. Now we think we are having a good life, and you think you have figured life out when things don't go wrong. However, when things start to go wrong, we seem to get a little lost, and over time it leads to frustration. This frustration will eventually lead to anger. Without balance in your life, most people are ill-equipped to deal with that anger without giving up on achieving their goals.

Greed can be a drug just like any substance because it creates a false sense of pleasure. Like any drug, greed can be addictive in nature. It can really be destructive to the body if not kept in check. What makes greed so hard to step away from is that it is enforced by our culture.

Most of us think about what we want more so than we think about what we need. "I want a nice car. I want a nice house. I want to get married." You get the message. But most people can't tell you why they want what they want. What makes our wants so important? What constitutes our sacrifice as worthy? Our value structure is based off of vanity, greed, and gluttony. We want far more than we need, and we can't wait to show it off once you have it. So is it any wonder that most people aren't happy because they spend their days living a lie?

We live our lives on many different levels and our value structure can sometimes reflect those levels. How we deal with sin and the right and wrong of things are examples of this. We as a people can overlook many things because of how we view the sin in our lives. If you were born into sin, wouldn't it make sense to see sin as an acceptable norm? (Everybody is doing it, so it can't be that bad right?)

Any one of these questions will spark a sense of truth in you about your life and if it's moving in the right direction. Can you change what you believe? If you have grown up your whole life believing the sky is blue, what would it take to change your mind? Would it take a day or maybe a month for you to believe that the sky was no longer blue? This example is to help explain how deep our beliefs about our lifestyles are ingrained in us. We are products of our environments. How many things do we take at face value because that is what someone else defined for you?

Today's Action Point: We are creatures of habit, and in our minds we say, "this is what I am used to." Is what you want based on what is best for you? Answer the following questions-- are you balanced? Happy? Healthy? Are your answers enough reason to want to start over?

DON'T BE SCARED TO TRY NEW THINGS; THAT'S WHAT STARTING OVER IS ALL ABOUT.

The kind of life you want to have will depend on what you consider to be of value to you. From an oppressed, reactive view of things, we don't seem to value our lives very much. Obesity is on the rise. Fast food makes billions. Healthy food costs too much. Water is toxic. Air is polluted, and people just don't care.

With these negative truths, don't you think starting over is the way to go? Doesn't it make sense to quit playing a victim and begin to take control of your life?

See life in a new way — learn to feel better, be happy, be and feel strong, and demand better from your world.

When people look to make major changes in their lives, normally they would hit rock bottom (like an alcoholic taking step 1 in an AA meeting — finally admitting to the problem). But beginning the journey to a healthy lifestyle can easily become a matter of perception. You don't have to wait to have a heart attack to change your ways! (Please don't wait until you have heart attack. If you've had a heart attack, then let's talk about making some changes.) You do not have to be obese or overweight to be unhealthy. A life filled with the wrong choices (such as stressing too much, moving too little, or overindulging in alcohol) can make you unhealthy as well. So don't get hung up on where you've been, but get focused on where you want to go.

Today's Action Step: Don't fear what you don't understand. What is holding you back from being your healthiest you? Learn what you don't understand and remove the fear road block on your journey to success.

DON'T BE BLINDED BY THE WORLD'S INFUENCES. BE POSITIVE ABOUT THE DECISIONS YOU MAKE. IF IT IS RIGHT, DO IT; IF IT IS WRONG, LET IT GO.

Being healthy is freedom. It gives you options; it lets you understand what is important in life. It will show you which way is up. To be unhealthy is to not understand what life can truly be like. It will seem like nothing is for you when you are not living in health, and you're always the last person to figure it out.

Have you ever thought what is it about your current life that keeps you from seeing the positive side of health and happiness? Why don't we pursue the good as much as we pursue the bad things in our life? Why are alcohol and sports celebrated while healthy eating and sports are not? Athletes don't drink while playing sports. Alcohol doesn't help the body in any meaningful way, but you can find commercials promoting alcoholic beverages during every nationally or regionally aired sporting event.

Our definition of fun is painted by society. You can't have any fun without a certain level of negative influences being invited to the party. Things like alcohol, eating fatty foods, and smoking tobacco are ingrained in the very fabric of American culture. The alarming reality is that it is a rite of passage to have negative influences in our lives in order to be accepted in our peer groups.

Here is a crazy way to look at things: if your mind can play tricks on you, how would you know if you're making the right choices? We know we second guess ourselves all the time. There is an old saying that states "your first choice is the right choice." However, this statement only applies with multiple choice tests in school! If your life has been filled with misdirection, it is common for your first choice to be the wrong one when it comes to making healthy decisions.

Today's Action Step: Be honest with yourself — make a list of negative influences in your life. Make a decision regarding if you are willing to let them go. If you are, make an action plan that includes healthier actions in place of your negative influences. Seek the help of a life coach, support group, counselor, or medical health professional if you are unable to make and stick with your plan.

ACCEPT THAT FAILURE IS A NECESSARY PART OF LIFE.

A healthy lifestyle is a new education for most people. Most of the time, we don't know what goes on in terms of being healthy other than what we see on TV or read in magazines. We take our knowledge in bits and pieces, and we never get a full understanding.

Letting go of your old life habits will most likely be the hardest thing you will have to do when it comes to living a new, healthy lifestyle because you were comfortable in the old. You knew what you were getting out of your old life, even if it probably wasn't a whole lot of what you needed. But we can't keep doing the same thing expecting different results, right? That's insanity. (And you won't get a t-shirt for that, because this is real insanity).

Some people will believe that they are too old to change. They believe "That's just how life is, so why try?" Or they may start a change and find themselves unsuccessful with their initial action plan. If you were to look at some of the most successful people in the world, they will tell you that failing is part of life. How else will you know what works if you haven't had the experience of knowing what doesn't work?

Motivation or lack thereof can come in any form, so being fearless can help you overcome them. Looking for more out of life is one of the reasons we live. The old pursuit of happiness included the American Dream where we work harder to get more stuff. This American Delusion is one of the causes of depression and self-doubt. We look to live that dream in the easiest, fastest way we can, and if we don't get it, we feel like we have failed in life.

Today's Action Step: What is your most recent failure on your journey to a healthier lifestyle? What have you learned from this experience?

BE FEARLESS IN YOUR PURSUIT OF A HEALTHY AND NEW LIFE.

Understand there will always be obstacles in your life and that they can manifest themselves in many forms:

>Mind: self-doubt, fear, lack of knowledge
>
>Body: being overweight or obese, not having the physical capacity needed to achieve what you want
>
>Spirit: temptation, lack of faith

For God has not given us the spirit of fear, but of power, and of love, and of a sound mind (2 Timothy 1:7, KJV)

We are comprised of three components — Body, Mind, and Spirit which are interdependent on each other (two or more things needy of each other). Let's look at this from a spiritual viewpoint. The flesh (the body) is comprised of what our parents looked like, what we eat, and what we've done. It seeks to please only itself and is bound to this earth. All it knows is worldly things and pleasures. It doesn't seek to please God because it only worries about itself, because it has to (for example, if it's cold, you will get goose bumps; if you're hungry, your stomach tightens; you get the point).

The heart and will (spirit) always seeks to please God because it's God's image. It's the part of Him that He put in our make-up. God is in you. Greatness and divine purpose from the Most High has been put in you ON PURPOSE! The spirit rejoices in what is good always.

The mind (which houses images and views the world gives us) will always agree with what it is fed the most! What are you feeding into? Fear? Failure? Stop! Majority rules; if your body doesn't possess the capacity to complete certain tasks, it relies on your mind, or your conscious and subconscious thoughts, for sustenance. If your mind is filled with "I can't do it" or "I'll always look like this," then it will not be able to push pass the obstacle.

Unlike your mind which can be filled with unproductive, self-defeating thoughts, when your spirit speaks, it will only tell you what you can do. Renew your mind with your spirit! Undo anything that tells you what you can't do! Nothing to it but to do it! (Feel free to read this step twice; there's some quality food there!)

Today's Action Step: Realize that your mind, body, and spirit all need each other! You have to feed them in the spiritual and physical realms. What are you feeding into others? What are you feeding yourself? How does this translate into your current state of health?

MAKE YOUR OWN DREAMS: LIVE THE LIFE OF TRUE HAPPINESS AND TRUE WEALTH- - YOUR HEALTH.

You can like the life you're living, you can live the life you like… (Chicago, the musical)

The life you want can only come through change. You must look for a new life inside of you! Be the change you want to see. Change begins with you. So start the walk that reflects the new you.

What can you do right now? Where does the change begin and how does that change look to you? What does healthy living look like to you? Everyone has a different picture. Unfortunately some of us are influenced by the media, and healthy might not be a size two running in a two-piece, and it doesn't have to be! It will look how you want it to look based on what you know about you. We can only see what we know — change what we know and your life will change with it!

Today's Action Step: Look for realistic images of what health looks like. Start a folder with cutouts or a file folder on your computer with images. Try to diversify your images with different sizes, shapes, and activities.

YOU MUST BELIEVE IN YOU AND YOUR JOURNEY. GOD WILL HELP YOU AS LONG AS YOU OPEN YOUR MIND, BODY, AND SPIRIT TO HIS WILL.

Do you believe in you? Sadly people find it easier to believe in magic than to believe in themselves. Part of your success on this journey rests upon you believing in what you want for yourself and believing that it is attainable. A lot of people say they want it. Still, when it is time to make it happen, they come up with a laundry list of excuses that prevents them from not only completing the journey but also prevents them from even getting started. Believing in yourself is the spiritual part of your journey. Having faith in what God has given you to change allows you to believe God will help you help yourself. So you must believe you can succeed in your journey.

Your body is the first thing God has given you, so He is aware of his temple. When you choose to open your heart to God's will, He will help you see what is needed for your life and give you strength in your journey to keep going. You will also have discernment with your strength to see that the difficult part of the road does not last forever; you will see the end of your struggle and reap the benefits of your commitment.

Your strength and discernment will also allow you to see that you can't do it all alone. As selfish beings, we don't want people in the messy or difficult part of our lives. We keep them at a distance because we don't want others to know how weak we are. Still, you must understand you can't do it yourself because you don't know it all. So as you're writing your questions on what you want and breaking down your answers regarding how to get there, you can get help in the areas where you are weak. Just ask! This help will keep you on task without panicking, getting discouraged, or giving up.

Today's Action Step: Study the Biblical meaning of discernment and strength, and pray for these qualities. Suggested texts for discernment include Proverbs 15:21, Isaiah 11:2-3, Luke 11:9, Hebrews 4:12, and 1 Thessalonians 5:21. Suggested text for strength include Psalm 28:7, Psalm 73:26, Psalm 118:14, Isaiah 33:2, 1 Corinthians 1:25, and Philippians 4:13.

GET HELP AS YOU WALK THROUGH YOUR JOURNEY OF STARTING OVER-- YOU CAN'T DO IT ALONE.

We have to accept that we don't know what we are doing, so we must stop acting like we do. Starting over is about making new choices. Being humble should be one of those choices. Life can be complicated enough by itself, but to do it alone shows that you have not thought it through.

Life is all about change—change your thinking, change your body, and change your life. Sometimes, we have to have help with the voices in our heads (yes, we all hear voices!). These voices or thoughts that cycle in our minds govern our existence. Sometimes, we need help interrupting the cycle, and this help comes through the voices of people with greater wisdom and experience in our area of need. These people are able to speak positivity into our lives and help us realize where we may have broken or misinformed thought patterns.

Today's Action Step: Seek out people that can strengthen you by interrupting your negative, misinformed, and broken thought patterns such as a pastor, fitness coach, life coach, mentor, workout partner, or individual who has been successful with changing their own health.

MAKE A SYSTEM THAT WORKS FOR YOU. DON'T GRAB SOMEONE ELSE'S SYSTEM BECAUSE THEY ARE NOT YOU.

What's for you is for you.

Thou shalt not covet thy neighbor's life, spouse, or their health system (My interpretation of Exodus 20:17.)

No matter who you are in this world, everyone has a rhythm or habits that dictate their life. So you must get your head wrapped around the fact that you must have a system in place designed for and by you to better your life. Your system will help you create your healthy walk that people will be able to see and identify as something different because it's you! Your change will be evident to other people, and they will want to mimic your healthy walk!

Making changes in your life will set you apart from other people. What will make you different is your healthy walk. You are choosing to live a healthy life, and you are choosing to put the positive and not the negative in your life. This action alone will look different to people, and it should look different because you are different! Sin is an acceptable norm nowadays, so your deviation from that path should make you stick out. You should be just fine knowing that this too is a part of the plan.

You must accept that your life will be different than people around you. Your new path will give you new insight on why health is important and why you are living a better life. You should help other people see that their life can get better as well. Each one reach one, and each one teach one.

Action Step: Take a moment to reflect on and list what was once easy for you to do (alone or with others) that is no longer your style.

CREATE YOUR SYSTEM AS YOU GET A CLEARER PICTURE OF YOUR VISION OF YOUR NEW LIFE COMING TOGETHER.

How fast you go in your journey will depend on your mental clarity of your vision. Each change you make with a positive result is a piece of the puzzle. You can add to your system because you have proven that it works. And most important, you will like how it looks!

So now you can begin to move at a pace that makes you feel more confident in your efforts. Now you have a look about yourself that other people can see, and it's just not the physical; it's an inner glow that becomes evident within you. It will feel good and you will be able to realize that this healthy walk feels better than your previous walk. You, my friend are new and improved.

What is your system? What does your system look like and how do you use it? Does your system help you stay on task and keep you moving in the right direction? The thing that makes a system important is that it teaches you rhythm. Keeping your system the same way every day helps you build a habit, and your habit builds a lifestyle. Your lifestyle becomes your way of life.

Today's Action Step: Once you have started learning the real you and you have asked all your questions, what do you do next? Write out where your current life is and where you'd like your healthy life to be. Next, write at least one tangible goal that will bridge where you are to where you are going.

WORDS FROM THE AUTHOR

If this book has been helpful, please write a brief testimony of your success and post it to the Amazon review of this title. Your reviews are extremely helpful and are used to improve future editions of this work.

Sincerely,

Darrin Eaddy

APPENDIX-- Recipes for Starting Over

Following are healthy recipes that can be used to fuel your body while pleasing your palate along your journey to health. Our recipes are designed to reduce your sodium, sugar, and fat intake.

Breakfast Green Smoothie

1 cup spinach

½ medium banana, frozen

1 cup frozen cherries, strawberries, or mangos

1 cup water

2 tbsp of hemp protein

Blend on high until smooth. Drink immediately. (1 serving)

Veggie Omelet

½ cup egg substitute or two whisked eggs

2 tbsp diced onion

2 tbsp diced bell pepper

2 tbsp diced mushrooms

2 tbsp diced tomatoes

2 tbsp fat free shredded cheddar cheese

¼ tsp garlic powder

non-stick cooking spray

Coat a skillet with the nonstick cooking spray. Sauté vegetables on medium heat for two minutes. Remove veggies from pan and spray again. Add egg substitute and sprinkle with garlic powder. Once the egg bubbles on the edges, add veggies and cheese. Once the liquid yolk cooks, fold over into a half- moon. Cook on both sides for an additional 30 seconds. (1 serving)

Curried Cauliflower

1 tbsp canola oil

¾ cup chopped onion

¾ cup frozen green peas

1 head chopped cauliflower, chopped

1 tbsp curry power

2 tsp cumin

1/8 tsp pepper

1/8 tsp salt

Steam cauliflower. Heat canola oil in a large skillet. Add onion and sauté for one minute. Add remaining ingredients and stir until vegetables are coated with spices. Cook on medium heat for 10 minutes, stirring often. Serve over brown rice. (4 servings)

Southern Style Green Beans

1 lb. green beans

¼ tsp. liquid smoke

1 tsp. vinegar

¼ cup water

Add water to the pot and bring to a boil. Add all other ingredients. Cover and reduce heat. Cook for 8 minutes for bright, crisp, greens. (4 servings)

Asian Slaw

1/3 cup rice vinegar

½ cup sugar (or sucralose)

1 tbs. soy sauce

1 tbs. fresh ginger, minced

½ crushed red pepper

4 cups of cabbage, chopped

1 cup carrots, shredded

1 medium onion, quartered and thinly sliced

½ cup green bell peppers, chopped

To make the dressing, combine the first five ingredients in a small bowl and set side. Combine the remaining ingredients toss in dressing. Cover and chill in the refrigerator for at least one hour before serving. (6 servings)

Marinated Salmon

1 lb salmon

1 cup pineapple juice

1 tbsp soy

2 tbsp fresh ginger, minced

1tbsp canola oil

Preheat oven 350°. Combine the juice, soy and ginger. Place in a sealable gallon-sized bag and add salmon. Marinate for at least 30 minutes. Heat olive oil in pan over medium heat. Sear salmon fillets on both sides. Finish in oven for 20 minutes. (4 servings)

Chili

1 lb ground chicken, turkey, or 90% lean ground beef

2 medium onions, chopped

2 medium green bell peppers, chopped

2 cans Rotel tomatoes

2 cans pinto beans

6 tbsp chili seasoning

1 tsp garlic powder

½ tsp ground cumin

½ tsp oregano, crushed

½ tsp salt

1 bottle of beer

Brown the meat in a skillet. Drain cooked meat in a colander. In a large pot, sauté onions and peppers with a little juice from the tomatoes. Add the meat, tomatoes, beans, seasoning ingredients and beer. Simmer for one hour. (4 servings)

Mediterranean Turkey Burgers

1 lb ground turkey

½ cup spinach, finely chopped

½ cup feta cheese

1/3 cup sundried tomato, finely chopped

1 tsp garlic powder

¼ tsp black pepper

Combine all ingredients. Form into 4 patties. Grill over medium heat until well done (internal temperature of 165°F. (4 servings)

Chocolate Mousse

1 ½ cup fat-free half and half

One1.4 ounce package fat-free, sugar free instant chocolate pudding

One 8-oz tub frozen light whipped topping, thawed

½ tsp rum extract

1 cup sliced strawberries

Whip half-and-half, extract and pudding until thick. Let chill in refrigerator for 10 minutes. Fold in whipped topping. Divide into 4 individual servings. Top each serving with ¼ cup fresh strawberries. (4 servings)

Made in the USA
Columbia, SC
25 March 2024

33256509R00041